YOGA ASANAS CHART BOOK

YOGA ASANAS CHART BOOK CONTAINS 60 COMMON POSES, ORGANIZED INTO THE FOLLOWING SIX CATEGORIES: STANDING, SUPINE, SEATED, PRONE, KNEELING, OTHER.

IT CAN BE USED IN ONE, TWO OR ALL THREE OF THE FOLLOWING WAYS: MINI POSTER, BOOK, FLASH CARDS.

HOW TO USE

MINI POSTER - IF YOU WANT TO POST THIS CHART ON THE WALL, SIMPLY OPEN THE STAPLE IN THE MIDDLE OF THE BOOKLET AND REMOVE TWO PAGES THEN PIN TWO COPIES ON THE WALL (ONE FOR EACH SIDE).

BOOK - LEAVE ONE COPY IN THE BOOK AND STAND IT UP AS YOU DO YOUR YOGA PRACTICE OR USE IT AS A REFERENCE TO STUDY FROM OUTSIDE OF YOUR PRACTICE TIME.

FLASH CARDS - CUT THE FIGURES OUT AND MAKE FLASH CARDS OUT OF THEM.

The Mindful Word - 1120 Finch Ave. W. Unit 701-928, Toronto, Ontario, M3J 3H7, Canada

Visit us online at www.themindfulword.org

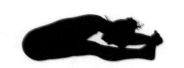

PASCHIMOTTANASANA
Seated Forward Bend

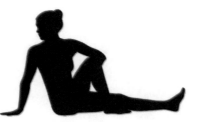

MARICHYASANA III
Marichi's Pose

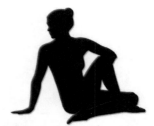

ARDHA MATYENDRASANA
Half Lord of the
Fishes Pose

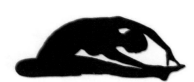

JANU SIRSASANA
Head-To-Knee Pose

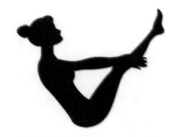

PARIPURNA NAVASANA
Boat Pose

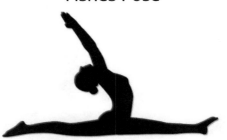

HANUMANASANA
Monkey Pose

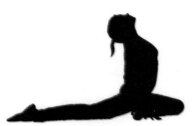

**EKA PADA
RAJAKAPOTASANA**
Pigeon Pose

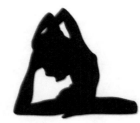

**EKA PADA
RAJAKAPOTASANA**
Pigeon Pose (variation)

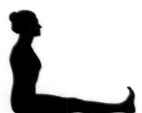

DANDASANA
Staff Pose

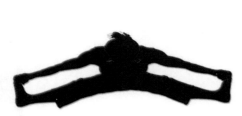

UPAVISTHA KONASANA
Wide-Angle Seated
Forward Bend

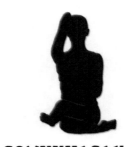

GOMUKHASANA
Cow Face Pose

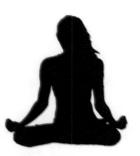

SVASTIKASANA
Cross Pose

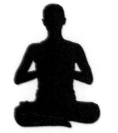

AGNISTAMBHASANA
Fire Log Pose

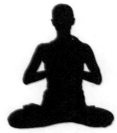
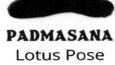

PADMASANA
Lotus Pose

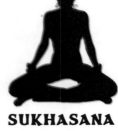

SUKHASANA
Easy Pose

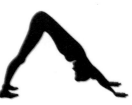

ADHO MUKHA SVANASANA
Downward-Facing Dog

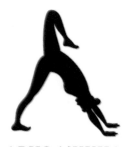

ADHO MUKHA SVANASANA
Downward-Facing Dog (variation)

UTTANA SHISHOSANA
Extended Puppy Pose

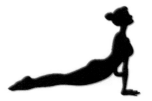

URDHVA MUKHA SVANASANA
Upward-Facing Dog

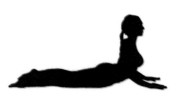

BHUJANGASANA
Cobra Pose

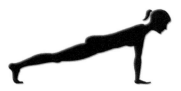

CHATURANGA DANDASANA
Four-Limbed Staff Pose

MAKARASANA
Crocodile Pose

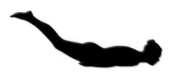

SALABHASANA
Locust Pose

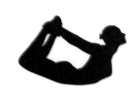

DHANURASANA
Bow Pose

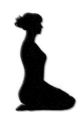

VAJRASANA
Thunderbolt Pose

BALASANA
Child's Pose

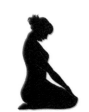

SIMHASANA
Lion Pose

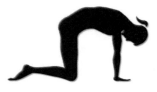

MARJARYASANA
Cat Pose

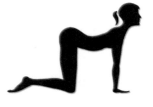

BITILASANA
Cow Pose

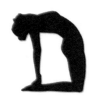

USTRASANA
Camel Pose

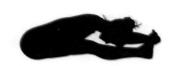

PASCHIMOTTANASANA
Seated Forward Bend

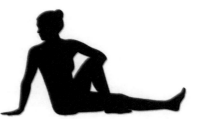

MARICHYASANA III
Marichi's Pose

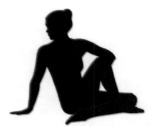

ARDHA MATYENDRASANA
Half Lord of the
Fishes Pose

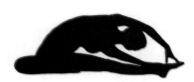

JANU SIRSASANA
Head-To-Knee Pose

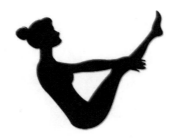

PARIPURNA NAVASANA
Boat Pose

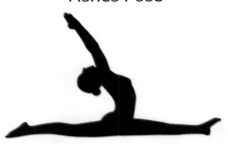

HANUMANASANA
Monkey Pose

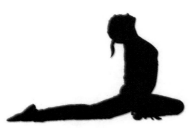

**EKA PADA
RAJAKAPOTASANA**
Pigeon Pose

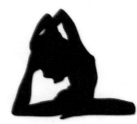

**EKA PADA
RAJAKAPOTASANA**
Pigeon Pose (variation)

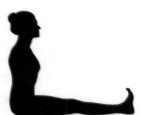

DANDASANA
Staff Pose

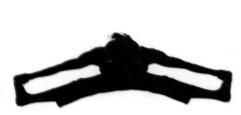

UPAVISTHA KONASANA
Wide-Angle Seated
Forward Bend

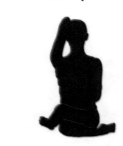

GOMUKHASANA
Cow Face Pose

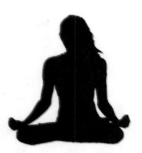

SVASTIKASANA
Cross Pose

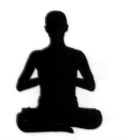

AGNISTAMBHASANA
Fire Log Pose

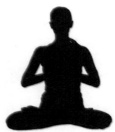
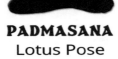

PADMASANA
Lotus Pose

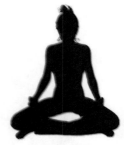

SUKHASANA
Easy Pose

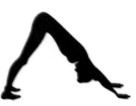

ADHO MUKHA SVANASANA
Downward-Facing Dog

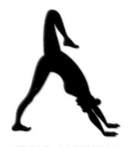

ADHO MUKHA SVANASANA
Downward-Facing Dog (variation)

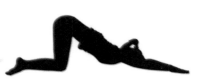

UTTANA SHISHOSANA
Extended Puppy Pose

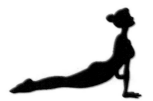

URDHVA MUKHA SVANASANA
Upward-Facing Dog

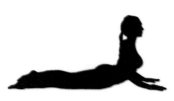

BHUJANGASANA
Cobra Pose

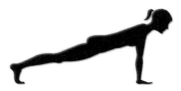

CHATURANGA DANDASANA
Four-Limbed Staff Pose

MAKARASANA
Crocodile Pose

SALABHASANA
Locust Pose

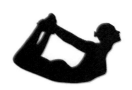

DHANURASANA
Bow Pose

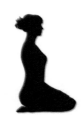

VAJRASANA
Thunderbolt Pose

BALASANA
Child's Pose

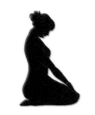

SIMHASANA
Lion Pose

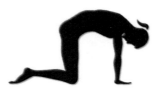

MARJARYASANA
Cat Pose

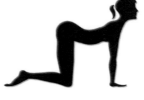

BITILASANA
Cow Pose

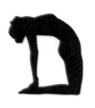

USTRASANA
Camel Pose

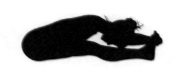

PASCHIMOTTANASANA
Seated Forward Bend

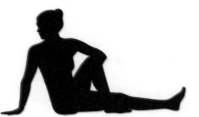

MARICHYASANA III
Marichi's Pose

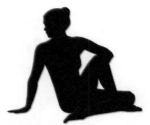

ARDHA MATYENDRASANA
Half Lord of the
Fishes Pose

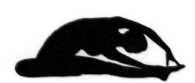

JANU SIRSASANA
Head-To-Knee Pose

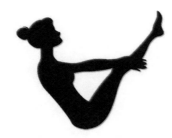

PARIPURNA NAVASANA
Boat Pose

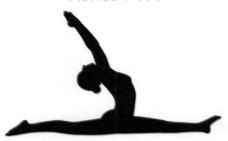

HANUMANASANA
Monkey Pose

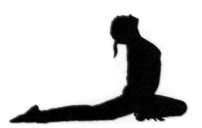

**EKA PADA
RAJAKAPOTASANA**
Pigeon Pose

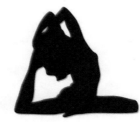

**EKA PADA
RAJAKAPOTASANA**
Pigeon Pose (variation)

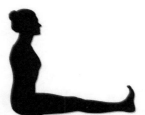

DANDASANA
Staff Pose

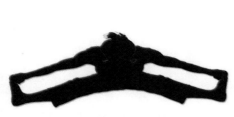

UPAVISTHA KONASANA
Wide-Angle Seated
Forward Bend

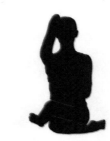

GOMUKHASANA
Cow Face Pose

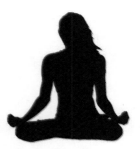

SVASTIKASANA
Cross Pose

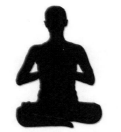

AGNISTAMBHASANA
Fire Log Pose

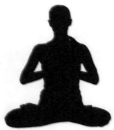

PADMASANA
Lotus Pose

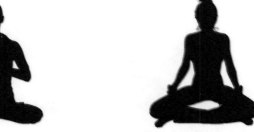

SUKHASANA
Easy Pose

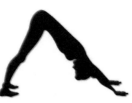

ADHO MUKHA SVANASANA
Downward-Facing Dog

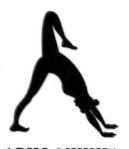

ADHO MUKHA SVANASANA
Downward-Facing Dog (variation)

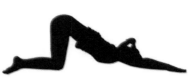

UTTANA SHISHOSANA
Extended Puppy Pose

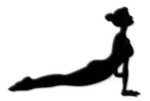

URDHVA MUKHA SVANASANA
Upward-Facing Dog

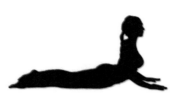

BHUJANGASANA
Cobra Pose

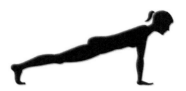

CHATURANGA DANDASANA
Four-Limbed Staff Pose

MAKARASANA
Crocodile Pose

SALABHASANA
Locust Pose

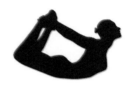

DHANURASANA
Bow Pose

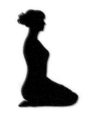

VAJRASANA
Thunderbolt Pose

BALASANA
Child's Pose

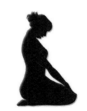

SIMHASANA
Lion Pose

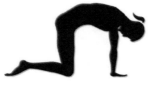

MARJARYASANA
Cat Pose

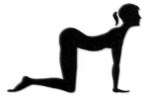

BITILASANA
Cow Pose

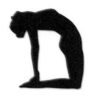

USTRASANA
Camel Pose

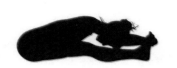

PASCHIMOTTANASANA
Seated Forward Bend

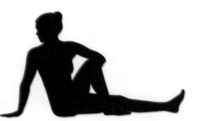

MARICHYASANA III
Marichi's Pose

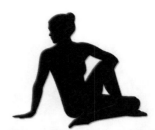

ARDHA MATYENDRASANA
Half Lord of the
Fishes Pose

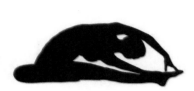

JANU SIRSASANA
Head-To-Knee Pose

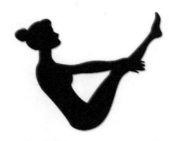

PARIPURNA NAVASANA
Boat Pose

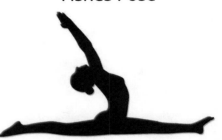

HANUMANASANA
Monkey Pose

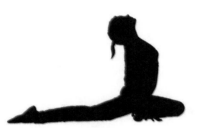

**EKA PADA
RAJAKAPOTASANA**
Pigeon Pose

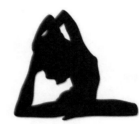

**EKA PADA
RAJAKAPOTASANA**
Pigeon Pose (variation)

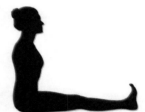

DANDASANA
Staff Pose

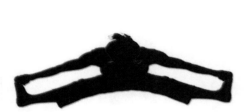

UPAVISTHA KONASANA
Wide-Angle Seated
Forward Bend

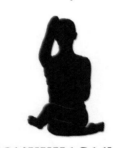

GOMUKHASANA
Cow Face Pose

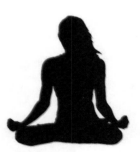

SVASTIKASANA
Cross Pose

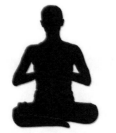

AGNISTAMBHASANA
Fire Log Pose

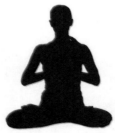

PADMASANA
Lotus Pose

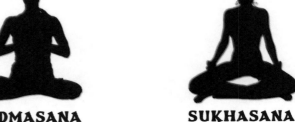

SUKHASANA
Easy Pose

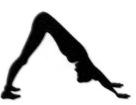

ADHO MUKHA SVANASANA
Downward-Facing Dog

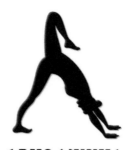

ADHO MUKHA SVANASANA
Downward-Facing Dog (variation)

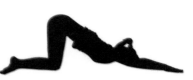

UTTANA SHISHOSANA
Extended Puppy Pose

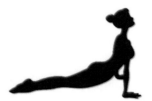

URDHVA MUKHA SVANASANA
Upward-Facing Dog

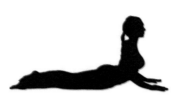

BHUJANGASANA
Cobra Pose

CHATURANGA DANDASANA
Four-Limbed Staff Pose

MAKARASANA
Crocodile Pose

SALABHASANA
Locust Pose

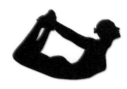

DHANURASANA
Bow Pose

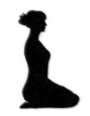

VAJRASANA
Thunderbolt Pose

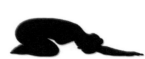

BALASANA
Child's Pose

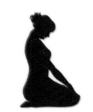

SIMHASANA
Lion Pose

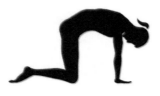

MARJARYASANA
Cat Pose

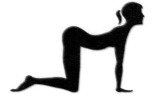

BITILASANA
Cow Pose

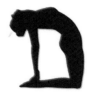

USTRASANA
Camel Pose

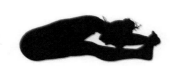

PASCHIMOTTANASANA
Seated Forward Bend

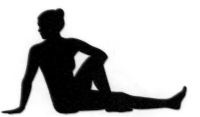

MARICHYASANA III
Marichi's Pose

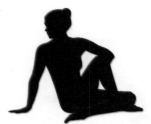

ARDHA MATYENDRASANA
Half Lord of the
Fishes Pose

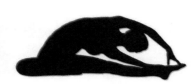

JANU SIRSASANA
Head-To-Knee Pose

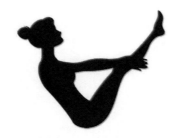

PARIPURNA NAVASANA
Boat Pose

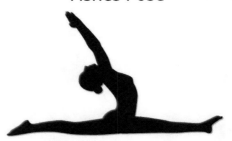

HANUMANASANA
Monkey Pose

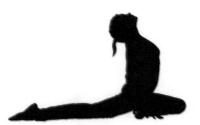

**EKA PADA
RAJAKAPOTASANA**
Pigeon Pose

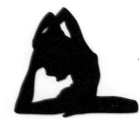

**EKA PADA
RAJAKAPOTASANA**
Pigeon Pose (variation)

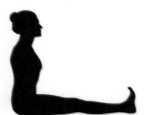

DANDASANA
Staff Pose

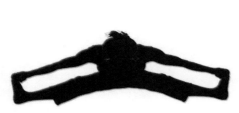

UPAVISTHA KONASANA
Wide-Angle Seated
Forward Bend

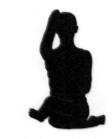

GOMUKHASANA
Cow Face Pose

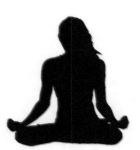

SVASTIKASANA
Cross Pose

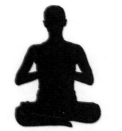

AGNISTAMBHASANA
Fire Log Pose

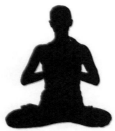

PADMASANA
Lotus Pose

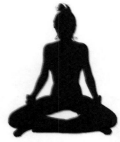

SUKHASANA
Easy Pose

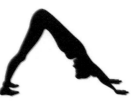

ADHO MUKHA SVANASANA
Downward-Facing Dog

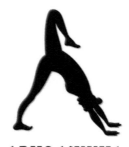

ADHO MUKHA SVANASANA
Downward-Facing Dog (variation)

UTTANA SHISHOSANA
Extended Puppy Pose

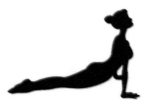

URDHVA MUKHA SVANASANA
Upward-Facing Dog

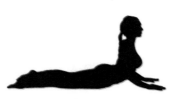

BHUJANGASANA
Cobra Pose

CHATURANGA DANDASANA
Four-Limbed Staff Pose

MAKARASANA
Crocodile Pose

SALABHASANA
Locust Pose

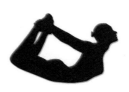

DHANURASANA
Bow Pose

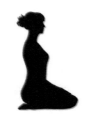

VAJRASANA
Thunderbolt Pose

BALASANA
Child's Pose

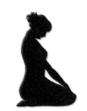

SIMHASANA
Lion Pose

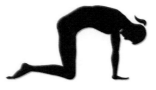

MARJARYASANA
Cat Pose

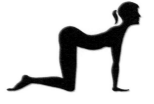

BITILASANA
Cow Pose

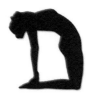

USTRASANA
Camel Pose

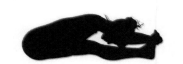

PASCHIMOTTANASANA
Seated Forward Bend

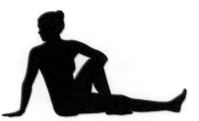

MARICHYASANA III
Marichi's Pose

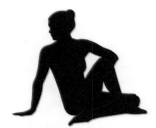

ARDHA MATYENDRASANA
Half Lord of the
Fishes Pose

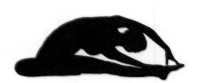

JANU SIRSASANA
Head-To-Knee Pose

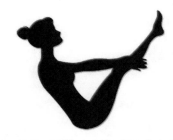

PARIPURNA NAVASANA
Boat Pose

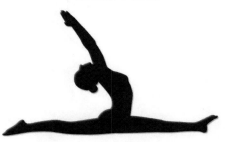

HANUMANASANA
Monkey Pose

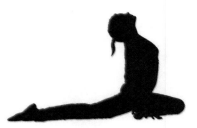

**EKA PADA
RAJAKAPOTASANA**
Pigeon Pose

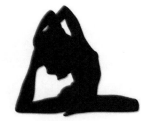

**EKA PADA
RAJAKAPOTASANA**
Pigeon Pose (variation)

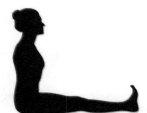

DANDASANA
Staff Pose

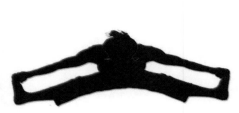

UPAVISTHA KONASANA
Wide-Angle Seated
Forward Bend

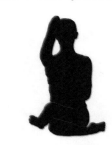

GOMUKHASANA
Cow Face Pose

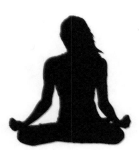

SVASTIKASANA
Cross Pose

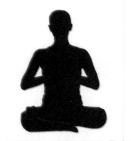

AGNISTAMBHASANA
Fire Log Pose

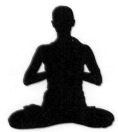
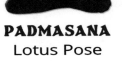

PADMASANA
Lotus Pose

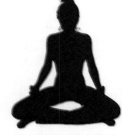

SUKHASANA
Easy Pose

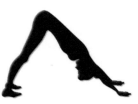

ADHO MUKHA SVANASANA
Downward-Facing Dog

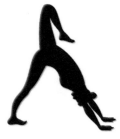

ADHO MUKHA SVANASANA
Downward-Facing Dog (variation)

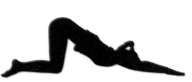

UTTANA SHISHOSANA
Extended Puppy Pose

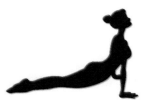

URDHVA MUKHA SVANASANA
Upward-Facing Dog

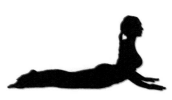

BHUJANGASANA
Cobra Pose

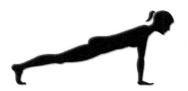

CHATURANGA DANDASANA
Four-Limbed Staff Pose

MAKARASANA
Crocodile Pose

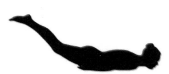

SALABHASANA
Locust Pose

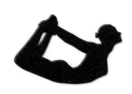

DHANURASANA
Bow Pose

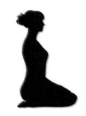

VAJRASANA
Thunderbolt Pose

BALASANA
Child's Pose

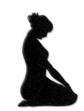

SIMHASANA
Lion Pose

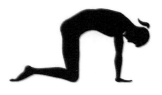

MARJARYASANA
Cat Pose

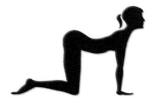

BITILASANA
Cow Pose

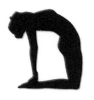

USTRASANA
Camel Pose

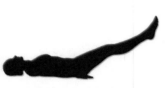

UTTANPADASANA
Raised-Leg Pose

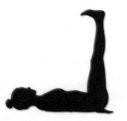

VIPARITA KARANI
Legs-Up-the-
Wall Pose

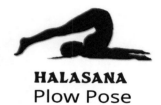

HALASANA
Plow Pose

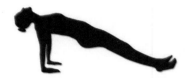

PAVANAMUKTASANA
Wind Liberating
Pose

MATSYASANA
Fish Pose

SAVASANA
Corpse Pose

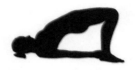

PURVOTTANASANA
Upward Plank Pose

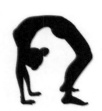

**SETU BANDHA
SARVANGASANA**
Bridge Pose

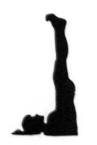

CHAKRASANA
Wheel Pose

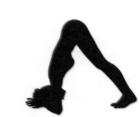

SARVANGASANA
Shoulderstand

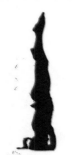

ARDHA SIRSASANA
Half Headstand

SIRSASANA
Headstand

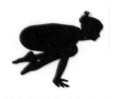

BAKASANA
Crow Pose

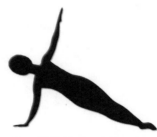

VASISTHASANA
Side Plank Pose

MALASANA
Garland Pose

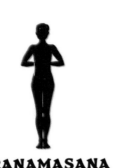

PRANAMASANA
Prayer Pose

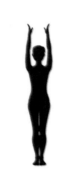

TALASANA
Palm Tree Pose

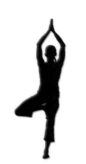

VRKSASANA
Tree Pose

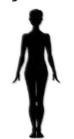

TADASANA
Mountain Pose

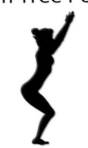

UTKATASANA
Chair Pose

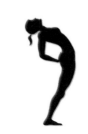

ANUVITTASANA
Standing Backbend Pose

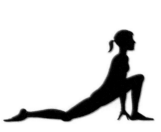

ANJANEYASANA
Low Lunge

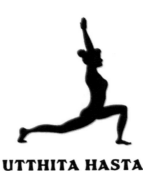

UTTHITA HASTA PADANGUSTASANA
High Lunge
(Crescent Variation)

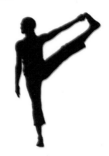

UTTHITA ASHVA SANCHALANASANA
Extended Hand-
To-Big-Toe Pose

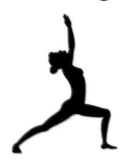

VIRABHADRASANA I
Warrior I Pose

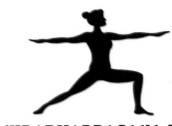

VIRABHADRASANA II
Warrior II Pose

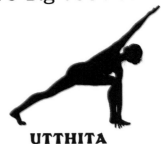

UTTHITA PARSVAKONASANA
Extended Side
Angle Pose

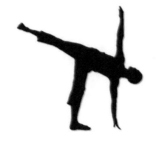

ARDHA CHANDRASANA
Half Moon Pose

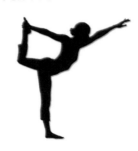

NATARAJASANA
Dancer's Pose

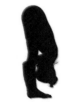

UTTANASANA
Standing Forward Bend

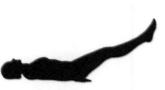

UTTANPADASANA
Raised-Leg Pose

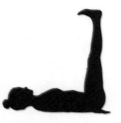

VIPARITA KARANI
Legs-Up-the-
Wall Pose

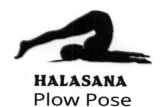

HALASANA
Plow Pose

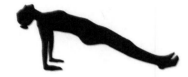

PAVANAMUKTASANA
Wind Liberating
Pose

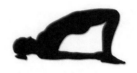

MATSYASANA
Fish Pose

SAVASANA
Corpse Pose

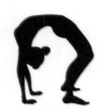

PURVOTTANASANA
Upward Plank Pose

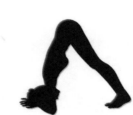

**SETU BANDHA
SARVANGASANA**
Bridge Pose

CHAKRASANA
Wheel Pose

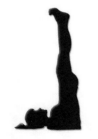

SARVANGASANA
Shoulderstand

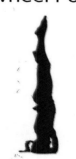

ARDHA SIRSASANA
Half Headstand

SIRSASANA
Headstand

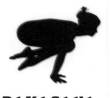

BAKASANA
Crow Pose

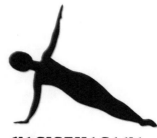

VASISTHASANA
Side Plank Pose

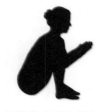

MALASANA
Garland Pose

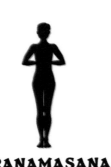

PRANAMASANA
Prayer Pose

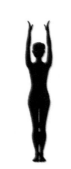

TALASANA
Palm Tree Pose

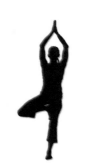

VRKSASANA
Tree Pose

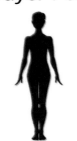

TADASANA
Mountain Pose

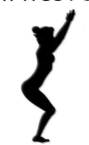

UTKATASANA
Chair Pose

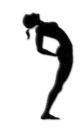

ANUVITTASANA
Standing Backbend Pose

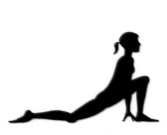

ANJANEYASANA
Low Lunge

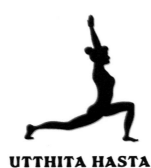

**UTTHITA HASTA
PADANGUSTASANA**
High Lunge
(Crescent Variation)

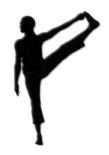

**UTTHITA ASHVA
SANCHALANASANA**
Extended Hand-
To-Big-Toe Pose

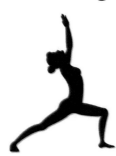

VIRABHADRASANA I
Warrior I Pose

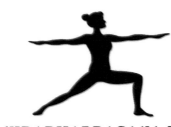

VIRABHADRASANA II
Warrior II Pose

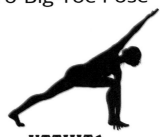

**UTTHITA
PARSVAKONASANA**
Extended Side
Angle Pose

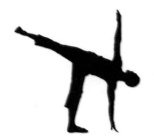

ARDHA CHANDRASANA
Half Moon Pose

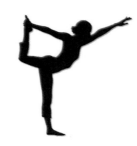

NATARAJASANA
Dancer's Pose

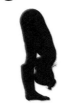

UTTANASANA
Standing Forward Bend

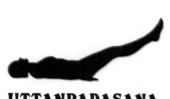

UTTANPADASANA
Raised-Leg Pose

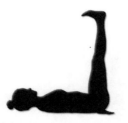

VIPARITA KARANI
Legs-Up-the-
Wall Pose

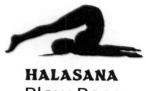

HALASANA
Plow Pose

PAVANAMUKTASANA
Wind Liberating
Pose

MATSYASANA
Fish Pose

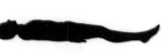

SAVASANA
Corpse Pose

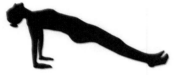

PURVOTTANASANA
Upward Plank Pose

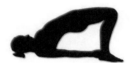

**SETU BANDHA
SARVANGASANA**
Bridge Pose

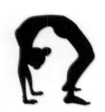

CHAKRASANA
Wheel Pose

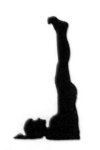

SARVANGASANA
Shoulderstand

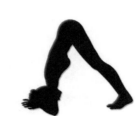

ARDHA SIRSASANA
Half Headstand

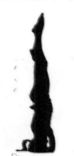

SIRSASANA
Headstand

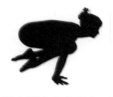

BAKASANA
Crow Pose

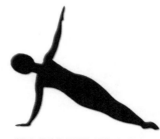

VASISTHASANA
Side Plank Pose

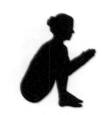

MALASANA
Garland Pose

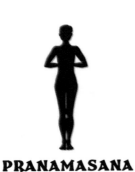

PRANAMASANA
Prayer Pose

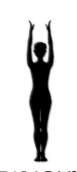

TALASANA
Palm Tree Pose

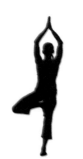

VRKSASANA
Tree Pose

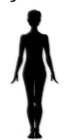

TADASANA
Mountain Pose

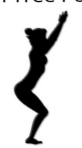

UTKATASANA
Chair Pose

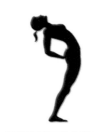

ANUVITTASANA
Standing Backbend Pose

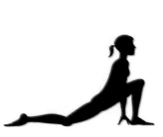

ANJANEYASANA
Low Lunge

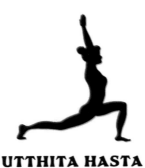

UTTHITA HASTA PADANGUSTASANA
High Lunge
(Crescent Variation)

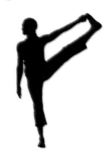

UTTHITA ASHVA SANCHALANASANA
Extended Hand-To-Big-Toe Pose

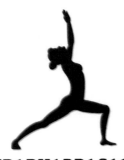

VIRABHADRASANA I
Warrior I Pose

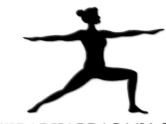

VIRABHADRASANA II
Warrior II Pose

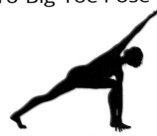

UTTHITA PARSVAKONASANA
Extended Side Angle Pose

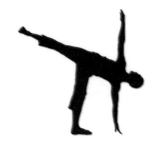

ARDHA CHANDRASANA
Half Moon Pose

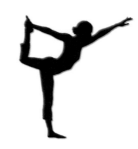

NATARAJASANA
Dancer's Pose

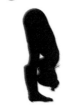

UTTANASANA
Standing Forward Bend

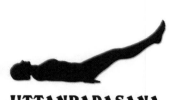

UTTANPADASANA
Raised-Leg Pose

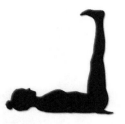

VIPARITA KARANI
Legs-Up-the-
Wall Pose

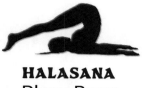

HALASANA
Plow Pose

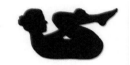

PAVANAMUKTASANA
Wind Liberating
Pose

MATSYASANA
Fish Pose

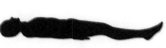

SAVASANA
Corpse Pose

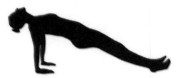

PURVOTTANASANA
Upward Plank Pose

**SETU BANDHA
SARVANGASANA**
Bridge Pose

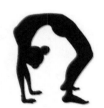

CHAKRASANA
Wheel Pose

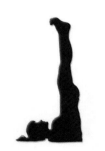

SARVANGASANA
Shoulderstand

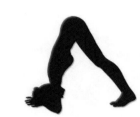

ARDHA SIRSASANA
Half Headstand

SIRSASANA
Headstand

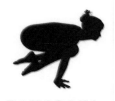

BAKASANA
Crow Pose

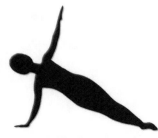

VASISTHASANA
Side Plank Pose

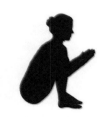

MALASANA
Garland Pose

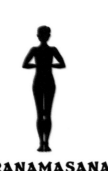

PRANAMASANA
Prayer Pose

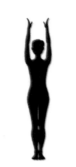

TALASANA
Palm Tree Pose

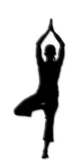

VRKSASANA
Tree Pose

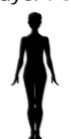

TADASANA
Mountain Pose

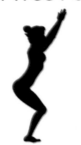

UTKATASANA
Chair Pose

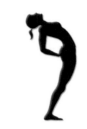

ANUVITTASANA
Standing Backbend Pose

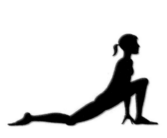

ANJANEYASANA
Low Lunge

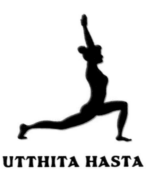

**UTTHITA HASTA
PADANGUSTASANA**
High Lunge
(Crescent Variation)

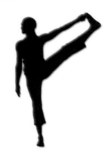

**UTTHITA ASHVA
SANCHALANASANA**
Extended Hand-
To-Big-Toe Pose

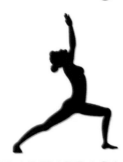

VIRABHADRASANA I
Warrior I Pose

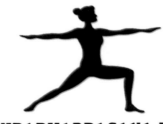

VIRABHADRASANA II
Warrior II Pose

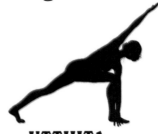

**UTTHITA
PARSVAKONASANA**
Extended Side
Angle Pose

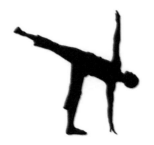

ARDHA CHANDRASANA
Half Moon Pose

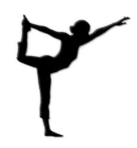

NATARAJASANA
Dancer's Pose

UTTANASANA
Standing Forward Bend

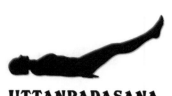

UTTANPADASANA
Raised-Leg Pose

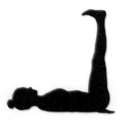

VIPARITA KARANI
Legs-Up-the-
Wall Pose

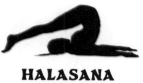

HALASANA
Plow Pose

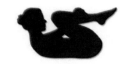

PAVANAMUKTASANA
Wind Liberating
Pose

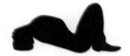

MATSYASANA
Fish Pose

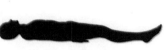

SAVASANA
Corpse Pose

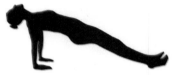

PURVOTTANASANA
Upward Plank Pose

**SETU BANDHA
SARVANGASANA**
Bridge Pose

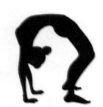

CHAKRASANA
Wheel Pose

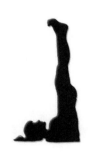

SARVANGASANA
Shoulderstand

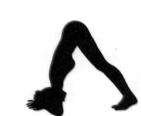

ARDHA SIRSASANA
Half Headstand

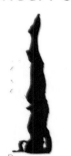

SIRSASANA
Headstand

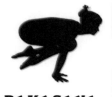

BAKASANA
Crow Pose

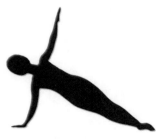

VASISTHASANA
Side Plank Pose

MALASANA
Garland Pose

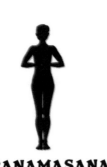

PRANAMASANA
Prayer Pose

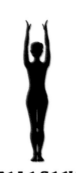

TALASANA
Palm Tree Pose

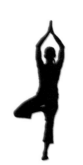

VRKSASANA
Tree Pose

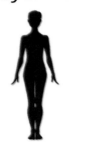

TADASANA
Mountain Pose

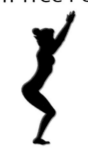

UTKATASANA
Chair Pose

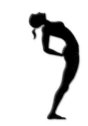

ANUVITTASANA
Standing Backbend Pose

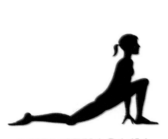

ANJANEYASANA
Low Lunge

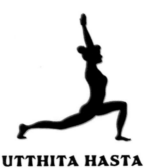

**UTTHITA HASTA
PADANGUSTASANA**
High Lunge
(Crescent Variation)

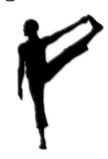

**UTTHITA ASHVA
SANCHALANASANA**
Extended Hand-
To-Big-Toe Pose

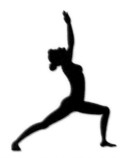

VIRABHADRASANA I
Warrior I Pose

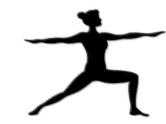

VIRABHADRASANA II
Warrior II Pose

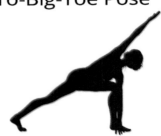

**UTTHITA
PARSVAKONASANA**
Extended Side
Angle Pose

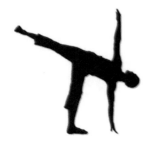

ARDHA CHANDRASANA
Half Moon Pose

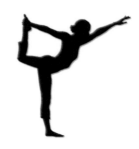

NATARAJASANA
Dancer's Pose

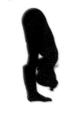

UTTANASANA
Standing Forward Bend

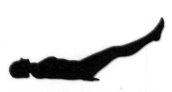

UTTANPADASANA
Raised-Leg Pose

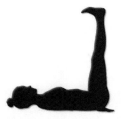

VIPARITA KARANI
Legs-Up-the-
Wall Pose

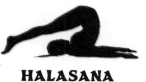

HALASANA
Plow Pose

PAVANAMUKTASANA
Wind Liberating
Pose

MATSYASANA
Fish Pose

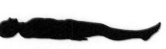

SAVASANA
Corpse Pose

PURVOTTANASANA
Upward Plank Pose

**SETU BANDHA
SARVANGASANA**
Bridge Pose

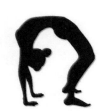

CHAKRASANA
Wheel Pose

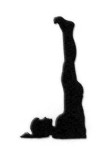

SARVANGASANA
Shoulderstand

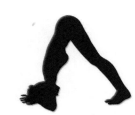

ARDHA SIRSASANA
Half Headstand

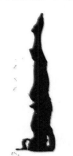

SIRSASANA
Headstand

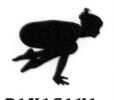

BAKASANA
Crow Pose

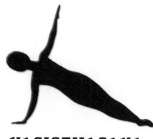

VASISTHASANA
Side Plank Pose

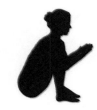

MALASANA
Garland Pose

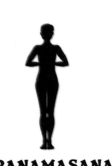

PRANAMASANA
Prayer Pose

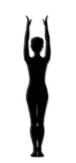

TALASANA
Palm Tree Pose

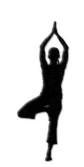

VRKSASANA
Tree Pose

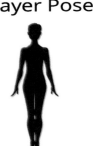

TADASANA
Mountain Pose

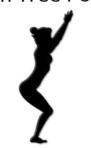

UTKATASANA
Chair Pose

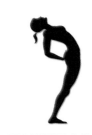

ANUVITTASANA
Standing Backbend Pose

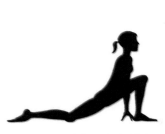

ANJANEYASANA
Low Lunge

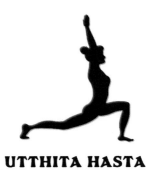

UTTHITA HASTA PADANGUSTASANA
High Lunge
(Crescent Variation)

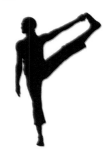

UTTHITA ASHVA SANCHALANASANA
Extended Hand-
To-Big-Toe Pose

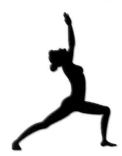

VIRABHADRASANA I
Warrior I Pose

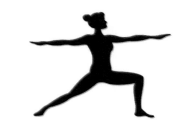

VIRABHADRASANA II
Warrior II Pose

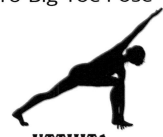

UTTHITA PARSVAKONASANA
Extended Side
Angle Pose

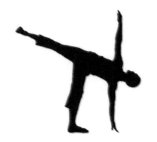

ARDHA CHANDRASANA
Half Moon Pose

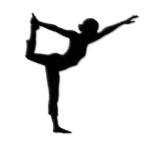

NATARAJASANA
Dancer's Pose

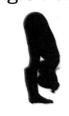

UTTANASANA
Standing Forward Bend

CPSIA information can be obtained
at www.ICGtesting.com
Printed in the USA
LVIC061539160819
627932LV00006B/29